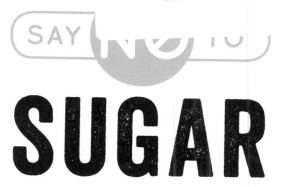

SAY NO TO

SUGAR

Simple Tips and Easy Recipes to Help You Cut Sugar Out of Your Life

Katherine Bassford

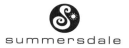

summersdale

SAY NO TO SUGAR

An Hachette UK Company
www.hachette.co.uk

Summersdale Publishers Ltd
Part of Octopus Publishing Group Limited
Carmelite House
50 Victoria Embankment
LONDON
EC4Y 0DZ
UK

www.summersdale.com

Printed and bound in Malta

ISBN: 978-1-78783-538-2

Substantial discounts on bulk quantities of Summersdale books are available to corporations, professional associations and other organizations. For details contact general enquiries: telephone: +44 (0) 1243 771107 or email: enquiries@summersdale.com.

CONTENTS

INTRODUCTION

When a fruit yogurt contains more sugar than ice cream, and a cereal bar is sweeter than chocolate, you know something's gone terribly wrong with our diets. Glance at the ingredients list of the food products you buy and you'll discover that sugar is everywhere. It lurks in everyday foods such as bread, soup, sauces and salad dressings – and it is used in gobsmacking amounts. A *Which?* analysis of 100 supermarket cereals found that almost two-thirds contained more sugar per recommended serving than a jam doughnut. (And, let's face it, who sticks to the suggested serving size? Research shows that most of us eat at least twice this amount.)

This book aims to put you back in control of your sugar intake, with as little stress as possible. It's purposefully slim on chemistry and big on the thing we're really interested in: the nuts and bolts of how to break a sugar addiction. "Addiction" may sound a little dramatic, but many of us are dependent on sugar to some degree or another, we just don't know it.

After getting to know why sugar is so bad for us, and how to spot it when it's hidden in so many foods, you'll find tips and tricks on breaking the sugar habit, reducing cravings and satisfying your sweet tooth naturally and healthfully. The low-sugar recipes at the end of the book will help make sure your new low-sugar or sugar-free day is still full of delicious meals and snacks to keep you well fed and energized.

Don't worry – you don't need to do all of this in one go. It's possible to achieve all of the above in small, easy steps...

THE SMALL-STEPS APPROACH

As a rule, extreme all-or-nothing goals and strict diets are recipes for failure. When it comes to lasting change, the only approach that works is something you can do each day and continue to do for the rest of your life.

In order to get yourself to do something you've been avoiding or find overwhelming, try taking a tiny step first – one so miniscule it's embarrassing! For example: to start exercising regularly, do one push up every day; to stop adding sugar to your cup of tea, remove a few grains from your teaspoon each week.

As ridiculous as it sounds, these tiny steps bypass the part of the brain (the amygdala) that triggers the fight or flight response whenever it senses danger (real or imagined). This allows you to tiptoe past fear and resistance and take one tentative step after another. You don't need a scientific study to tell you this approach works. Which are you more likely to do: cut out all sugar from this moment on, or buy one less can of fizzy drink a week?

Any behaviour that is repeated frequently lays down new neural pathways in the brain. Day by day, you are building new healthy-eating habits. Before you know it, you're doing the thing you previously thought you couldn't (even if it's something as simple as not adding sugar to your tea). The trick is to choose a first step that is so easy and non-threatening that you cannot fail. If you ever find yourself making excuses, cut back on the size of the step!

WHAT'S SO BAD ABOUT SUGAR?

We know too much sugar can make us overweight – that's a given – but it can also make us sick. Increasingly, the signs indicate that sugar, or – more specifically – fructose (table sugar is 50 per cent fructose), is the culprit behind rising levels of obesity worldwide and possibly a host of other illnesses, too, including heart disease and diabetes. This chapter is your crash course in what sugar actually is and why it's so bad for us.

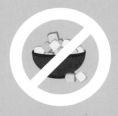

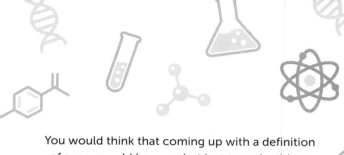

You would think that coming up with a definition of sugar would be easy, but just to make things difficult, there are several types of sugar, and what scientists call "sugar" and what we call "sugar" are two slightly different things:

- What we call sugar (the stuff we put in our food and in our hot drinks) is officially called sucrose.
- When scientists talk about "blood sugar", they are referring to glucose.

For the average person trying to learn about sugar, this is not spectacularly helpful. (It's also something food manufacturers are all too aware of and will exploit if you're not careful.) Thankfully, you don't need a PhD in biochemistry to understand sugar; you just need a few basic facts.

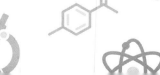

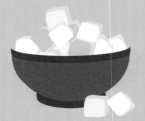

All sugars are carbohydrates.
"Carbohydrate" simply means molecules
made from carbon, hydrogen and oxygen.
There are several different types of sugar:
glucose, fructose ("fruit sugar"), sucrose ("table
sugar"), lactose ("milk sugar"), galactose (part
of lactose) and maltose ("malt sugar").
Don't worry about remembering all the
names. For the purpose of this book,
the sugars we're really interested in are
glucose, fructose and sucrose.

- Glucose is found naturally in plants
  (fruit, vegetables, beans and grains).
- Fructose is found naturally in fruit, honey
  and, to a lesser extent, vegetables.
- Sucrose is extracted from sugar cane
  and sugar beets; it contains 50 per cent
  glucose and 50 per cent fructose.

While we need glucose in order for our brain and body to function properly, we can get all of our daily glucose needs by eating a balanced diet. Glucose occurs naturally in fruit and vegetables. In addition, a proportion of the protein and fat we consume is changed into glucose once eaten. So, as far as the body is concerned, all natural food provides glucose. Not only is there no physiological requirement for sugars other than glucose in our diet, such sugars are actually toxic, especially in the unprecedented amounts we now eat.

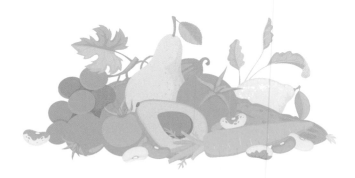

The World Health Organization (WHO)'s guidelines suggest that cutting the amount of sugar we eat from the current recommended limit of 10 per cent of our total calorie intake per day to 5 per cent would be beneficial. That's about 25 g, or 6 teaspoons, of sugar per adult per day. This is less than the amount of sugar found in one 50 g chocolate bar or can of fizzy drink.

This limit includes sugars added to food as well as sugars that are naturally present in honey, syrups, fruit juices and fruit concentrate. It does not include the sugars in fresh fruit, vegetables and milk.

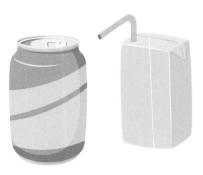

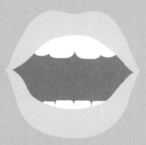

Americans consume 44 teaspoons of extra, non-naturally occurring sugar a day (68 kg, or 150 lb, a year), according to the US Department of Agriculture. Brits each consume more than 13 teaspoons a day on average, with some people consuming up to 46 teaspoons – that's an average of 411 g of added sugar a week, or nearly one small bag of sugar! Over 50 per cent of people around the world are overweight or obese, and over 400 million people have diabetes.

Soft drinks account for around 30 per cent of children's sugar intake. In the UK almost one quarter of five-year-olds suffer from tooth decay, and nearly 500 children a week are admitted to hospital with rotten teeth.

It's not just obviously sweet things
that we need to be wary of, though;
sugar is hiding in many everyday foods:

FOOD	ADDED SUGAR
Dollop of tomato sauce	**1–2** teaspoons
Cereal bar	**Up to 8** teaspoons
Serving of muesli	**Up to 4** teaspoons
Serving of pasta sauce from a jar	**2** teaspoons
Cinnamon latte	**6–7** teaspoons
Serving of berry-flavoured water	**5** teaspoons
Tin of soup	**3** teaspoons
Fruit smoothie	**6** teaspoons
Probiotic drink	**2** teaspoons
Flavoured yogurt	**4–6** teaspoons
Falafel wrap	**Up to 2** teaspoons

SIX REASONS TO AVOID SUGAR

We've grown up being told that sugar is bad for us because it contains "empty calories" and it's no friend to teeth. But that's just the tip of the iceberg. Evidence is mounting that excessive amounts of sugar wreak havoc on our metabolism and set us up for weight gain and many serious diseases. One sugar in particular seems to be especially bad for us. Fructose, found in table sugar and high fructose corn syrup, behaves in a way that is very different from any other sugar. This is what excessive sugar in our diet does to us...

Note: The following problems are essentially a dosage issue. Small doses of sugar, such as the natural sugar found in fruits, won't cause the health issues mentioned in this chapter. Large doses consumed over time (as found in a typical Western diet) can be highly toxic.

1. SUGAR MAKES US EAT MORE

Normally, appetite hormones signal to the brain when we've had enough to eat, but fructose doesn't play by the rules. It doesn't trigger "stop eating" hormones, so it sneaks in undetected. This explains why we can munch our way through a whole pack of sweets or crisps without feeling full.

It gets worse: fructose turns into fat in the body (see point 2), and fat interferes with our appetite control system. Hormones that normally tell us when to stop eating, such as cholecystokinin, insulin and leptin, no longer work as well as they should. Result: we feel hungry and end up eating more of every type of food, not just sugar!

2. SUGAR MAKES US OVERWEIGHT

Fructose is metabolized differently from glucose. Whereas glucose is used to fuel every cell in the body, most of the fructose we eat shoots straight to the liver where it is converted to fat (triglycerides). This fat either stays in the liver, where it can build up and cause non-alcoholic fatty liver disease (NAFLD), or it gets released into the bloodstream, increasing our risk of obesity, heart disease and stroke.

The worldwide obesity problem has been accelerating in direct proportion to our consumption of sugar. In the UK, one in four children is overweight or obese. In the US, it's around 30 per cent.

3. SUGAR CAUSES INSULIN RESISTANCE

During digestion, food and drink are broken down into glucose. In response to rising blood sugar levels, the pancreas secretes a hormone called insulin. Insulin acts like a key that unlocks the door into cells, such as muscle cells, so that glucose can be taken on as fuel. If we keep eating sugary food, the body tries desperately to keep up by producing more and more insulin. Eventually, the pancreas gets worn out and stops producing insulin, or our cells become numb to insulin and we become insulin-resistant. Result: elevated, and potentially toxic, blood sugar levels.

While further research is required before we can say that excess sugar actually causes type 2 diabetes, there is a strong correlation between countries that have the highest sugar consumption and the highest number of deaths from diabetes. Less than 30 years ago, type 2 diabetes was virtually unheard of. Now it affects 300 million people worldwide.

4. SUGAR RAISES YOUR RISK OF CHRONIC DISEASE

Excess sugar consumption is now thought to underlie many diseases prevalent in Europe and North America:

- A major US study conducted by the Harvard T.H. Chan School of Public Health in 2014 found that people who received more than a quarter of their daily calories through added sugar were almost three times more likely to die of cardiovascular disease than those who consumed less than a quarter of their calories from sugar.

- In a study published in the American Journal of Clinical Nutrition, drinking two or more fizzy or syrup-based drinks each day was linked to a 90 per cent added risk of developing pancreatic cancer.

- Studies show that consuming one sugary soft drink a day can raise your risk of diabetes and heart disease by 20 per cent.

5. SUGAR AFFECTS THE BRAIN

Sugar can also affect your emotions and mental health. The brain depends on an even supply of glucose to function. Excess sugar consumption has been linked to a wide range of psychological problems, including:

- Anxiety
- Depression
- Aggression
- Hyperactivity
- Impaired thinking
- Diminished attention span
- Problems concentrating
- Impaired memory and learning
- Dementia

Research into how sugar affects the brain is still in progress, but it's thought that sugar damages the brain's blood vessels and can cause brain shrinkage. In 2010, UCLA researchers discovered that the brains of overweight and obese people look between eight and 16 years older, and have less brain tissue, than the brains of those the same age and of healthy weight.

6. SUGAR IS ADDICTIVE

Eat a spoonful of chocolate cake and your brain will do a little happy dance. Sugar stimulates taste receptors on your tongue, which send a signal to the cerebral cortex in the brain. This triggers the release of dopamine, which makes us feel good – cue more chocolate cake. As having variety in our diet means we're more likely to get all the nutrients we need, the brain has evolved to pay special attention to new or different tastes. This means that if we eat sugary food day after day, less and less dopamine is released and we need more and more sugary food to get the same warm, fuzzy feeling. This is how sugar becomes addictive (some scientists say it's as addictive as cocaine). If you maintain a healthy, low-sugar diet and eat the odd piece of chocolate cake, it won't have the same effect.

SUGAR FROM GRAINS AND REFINED CARBOHYDRATES

For optimal health, you may want to consider reducing the amount of grains you eat, particularly if you usually eat them several times a day. Refined carbohydrates, such as crisps, crackers, bread, pasta, rice and cereal, have had much of their fibre and nutrients stripped away, meaning they are digested quickly and are rapidly converted to glucose. Unless you are very active and use up the excess glucose, these foods can raise blood sugar and insulin levels, promoting fat storage and other health problems associated with high blood sugar. Wholegrain versions are generally better options, though many have an impact on blood glucose levels that is similar to the refined "white" versions. For example, wholewheat bread spikes blood sugar just as quickly as white bread.

HELLO, SUGAR-FREE LIVING!

So, what benefits can you look forward to on your journey to low- or no-sugar living?

- Fewer (or no) cravings
- A clearer mind
- A more balanced mood
- Weight loss
- Younger-looking skin
- More restful sleep
- Reduced risk of tooth decay
- Reduced risk of developing health problems, including many chronic diseases

SUGAR FAQS

The topic of eating less sugar naturally triggers lots of questions. How far do you need to go with this? Which sweetener should you choose from the bewildering array? Should you switch to brown sugar? Is honey a better alternative? What about agave or artificial sweeteners? This chapter should help clear up any confusion.

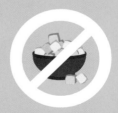

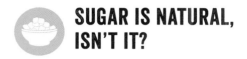

SUGAR IS NATURAL, ISN'T IT?

Table sugar is "natural" in the sense that it comes from a plant (sugar cane or sugar beet), but "natural" implies we are eating it in its unrefined state, which couldn't be further from the truth. Natural sugar from a sugar cane is passed through many systems and comes into contact with numerous chemicals to refine it into the white granules we add to our food and drink – stripping the natural vitamins and minerals along the way. Regardless of whether sugar is natural or not, there's one argument no one can quibble with: the amount of sugar in our diets is decidedly *unnatural*.

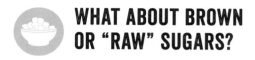 # WHAT ABOUT BROWN OR "RAW" SUGARS?

It's tempting to think that brown sugar is healthier than white sugar, but sadly this isn't the case. Brown sugar is either unrefined sugar which has some residual molasses in it, or it's a fake (i.e. it's really refined sugar which has had molasses added back in to give it an appealing colour and flavour). Dark brown sugar contains more molasses than light brown sugar, hence the difference in colour.

"Raw" sugars, such as light muscovado, dark muscovado and demerara, are not raw at all. They are partially refined, having been repeatedly boiled and crystallized to get a different concentration of molasses to produce the various colours. Molasses does contain nutrients, but the amount we're talking about is negligible. In summary, your body doesn't care; it's still sugar, and it will still have the same destructive effects.

HONEY'S FINE THOUGH, RIGHT?

This is where things get tricky. Honey tends to have slightly less of an effect on blood glucose levels than sugar. It also contains antioxidants, enzymes, vitamins and minerals, and has antibacterial and anti-inflammatory properties. The problem is, honey is 80 per cent sugar (fructose and glucose). Worse, its fructose content is 40 per cent. So in terms of fructose intake, there's really not much difference between eating a spoonful of table sugar and a spoonful of honey.

The jars of honey we buy from supermarkets are heavily processed and subject to excessive heating – to the point where honey's nutritional and medicinal properties are drastically reduced or have given up the ghost altogether.

If you decide to eat honey, go for raw honey (unfiltered and unheated) or unprocessed manuka honey and eat it sparingly. In general, darker honeys, such as buckwheat honey, contain more antioxidants than regular honey.

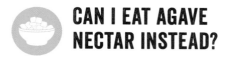# CAN I EAT AGAVE NECTAR INSTEAD?

Agave syrup is advertised as being "natural", but the reality is, it is highly processed, it has no health benefits and it is up to 90 per cent fructose – worse than table sugar and high fructose corn syrup.

You'll often see agave being touted as a "low-GI" sugar. The reason agave ranks low on the glycaemic index is because it contains so much fructose. Fructose, as we know, is not metabolized well by the body and goes straight to the liver, so it doesn't cause elevated blood glucose. For this reason, be extra wary of "low-GI" jams and spreads – the easiest way to make something low GI is to pack it full of fructose, often disguised as "grape concentrate".

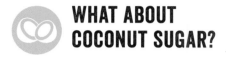

WHAT ABOUT COCONUT SUGAR?

Avoid high-sugar sweeteners such as golden syrup, commercial maple syrup, coconut sugar (coconut palm sugar), coconut syrup and coconut nectar. All are around 40 per cent fructose.

The reason raw coconut is fine to eat (i.e. flakes, flour, desiccated) is because it's the flesh of the coconut. Coconut sugar, syrup and nectar, on the other hand, are made from the sap of the coconut tree, which is boiled to create a syrup that is 70–80 per cent sucrose – half of which is fructose.

FRUIT'S HEALTHY, NO?

Fruit has health benefits, but it still contains very high levels of fructose (grapes, apples, pears, mangos, cherries and bananas are the worst offenders). But don't get too hung up on it! Fruit has been in our diets since the first humans evolved. We have evolved to process the fructose in fruit, just not in excessive amounts (i.e. not in conjunction with our modern-day high-sugar diets). If you have no blood sugar issues and are able to eat fructose without any digestive problems, then around two pieces of fruit a day is fine (one serving of fruit for an adult is around 80 g – one piece of tennis-ball-sized fruit or a handful of grapes). Fruit should be a supplement rather than the main part of your diet. In other words, avoid eating it for breakfast AND drinking juice AND snacking on dried fruit and fresh fruit throughout the day.

SO, WHAT'S THE BEST FRUIT TO EAT?

As you might have gathered, there is no conclusive answer. The one thing that most people seem to agree on is that, when you weigh up both nutrition and fructose content, berries come out on top.

Some fruits contain more vitamins and antioxidants than others. The health benefits of many fruits outweigh their high fructose content. Apples, for example, are rich in important antioxidants and fibre. Eating apples has been linked to lowering the risk of chronic diseases, including type 2 diabetes, cancer, heart disease and dementia.

Fibre content also varies a lot between fruits, and fibre-rich fruit breaks down more slowly in the body. A pear contains more fructose than an orange, but it also contains more fibre, so overall it's the better choice. The fruits with the lowest fructose content are apricots, kiwis, raspberries, strawberries, grapefruit, honeydew melon and lemons and limes.

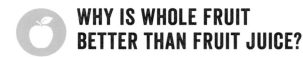

WHY IS WHOLE FRUIT BETTER THAN FRUIT JUICE?

Whole fruits are loaded with fibre, which slows down the rate at which sugar enters the bloodstream. The fructose in fruit bypasses our appetite control mechanisms, but the fibre makes us feel full and can help insulin do its work. All in all, nature has created a perfectly balanced package. The liver can easily metabolize small amounts of fructose (i.e. two pieces of fruit) without being overloaded. The proviso to this is: don't *drink* your fruit.

Drinking a glass of fruit juice is the equivalent of consuming several pieces of fruit in a short space of time, without the fibre. A glass of apple juice (freshly squeezed or otherwise) contains around 8 teaspoons of sugar, the same as a glass of cola. It also contains the same number of calories. To make matters worse, as there's no fibre or chewing to slow down consumption, it's easy to consume large portions of fruit juice and soft drinks very quickly.

However, it's not just the amount of sugar that's a concern. As fruit juice and a lot of soft drinks (e.g. squashes and fizzy drinks) are sugar in liquid form, large amounts of sugar hit the liver quickly and are converted into fatty acids, which can increase your risk of developing diabetes, cardiovascular disease and liver disease. Plus, you're bathing your teeth in sugar solution. Bacteria in our mouths feed off sugar and produce an acid. The longer the acid is in contact with the teeth, the worse the risk of tooth decay. The sugars in whole fruit are less likely to cause tooth decay because the sugar is contained within the structure of the fruit.

WHAT ABOUT DRIED FRUIT?

The reason dried fruit tastes so good is because it's 50–70 per cent sugar, a large proportion of which is fructose. Most dried fruit contains the same amount of sugar per fruit as the fresh version (though some have added sugar) – the issue is portion control. Dried fruit is less filling than fresh fruit due to its lack of water. Most of us would baulk at eating ten fresh apricots in one sitting, but we wouldn't think twice about eating ten dried ones. A handful of dates contains around 7 teaspoons of sugar, while sultanas, currants, dried cranberries and dried apples all have more than 60 per cent sugar content. A standard chocolate bar is around 60 per cent sugar, containing around 6 teaspoons of sugar.

WHAT'S HIGH FRUCTOSE CORN SYRUP (HFCS)?

High fructose corn syrup (also known as "glucose-fructose syrup" in the UK) is a highly sweet, gloopy syrup that is manufactured from corn syrup by converting a large proportion of its glucose into fructose. ("Corn syrup" is made from corn starch, and is 100 per cent glucose.) It's cheaper than sugar and extends the shelf life of products, which is why it can be found in most processed foods and drinks, cereal bars, doughnuts, chocolate bars, biscuits and ice cream.

HFCS is 55 per cent fructose and 42 per cent glucose (i.e. slightly higher in fructose than table sugar and with roughly the same fructose content as honey). The manufacture of HFCS also involves the use of artificial and synthetic agents, which may be harmful to health. It's also highly addictive. HFCS in diets has been linked to cardiovascular disease, diabetes and non-alcoholic fatty liver disease.

CAN I SWITCH TO ARTIFICIAL SWEETENERS INSTEAD?

Artificial sweeteners are several times sweeter than table sugar, so less is required to sweeten food, which sounds promising. However, they are relative newcomers to our diet, so we simply don't know whether they're safe for long-term consumption. The European Food Safety Authority (EFSA) assessed the evidence and concluded that aspartame, one of the compounds used as a sweetener, is safe and poses no threat to health "at current levels of exposure".

However, many scientists are still concerned and say artificial sweeteners may lead to:

- Weight gain
- Increased cravings for sugar
- Headaches and dizziness
- Depression
- Brain cancer
- Adverse effects on blood sugar and insulin levels

The four main artificial sweeteners are saccharin, cyclamate, aspartame (marketed as NutraSweet) and sucralose. You will frequently see them cropping up in carbonated soft drinks, especially "diet" versions.

Some manufacturers have switched to using sugar alcohols (a type of alcohol prepared from sugar) such as sorbitol, maltitol, mannitol and xylitol. Sugar alcohols do not cause tooth cavities, so they are often used in sugar-free gum. However, they affect blood sugar levels and, because they are not absorbed by the gut, can cause bloating and diarrhoea.

Sweeteners can be used to help wean yourself off sugary foods, but they are best used in small amounts and only for a short period of time. A study by the Harvard T.H. Chan School of Public Health has suggested that children should avoid artificially sweetened drinks altogether.

READING FOOD LABELS

With sugar present in so many supermarket products, there's a simple way to reduce the amount of sugar in your diet: avoid all processed food! Simple, but not necessarily easy. At the very least, sniff out the worst offenders and boot them from your basket. It takes seconds to read a food label once you get used to it, and you'll have the satisfaction of knowing you're taking your health and well-being into your own hands.

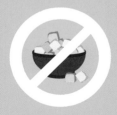

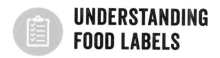

UNDERSTANDING FOOD LABELS

Food manufacturers are not legally required to specify the type of sugar in their products, so all we get to go by is a figure under the heading "carbohydrate (of which sugars)". When a label says "sugars", it's potentially referring to all types of sugar – naturally occurring (from fruit and milk) and added. That's why it's a good idea to resort to checking the ingredients list for anything nasty lurking there (see pp.42–43).

Look for the "per 100 g/ml" column and look at the "carbohydrate (of which sugars)" number. If the figure is 20 g per 100 g, for instance, the product is 20 per cent sugar.

If a food product contains less than 5 g of sugar per 100 g, it is considered to be low in sugar. If a product contains more than 15 g of sugar per 100 g, it is considered to be high in sugar.

HOW TO CALCULATE HOW MANY TEASPOONS OF SUGAR THERE ARE IN A SERVING

If you prefer to visualize how many teaspoons of sugar there are in a serving, you can work it out by dividing the number of grams of sugar in the "per serving" column by 4.2 (the weight of a teaspoon of sugar). If you don't have a calculator to hand, roughly divide the figure by four.

Bear in mind that a manufacturer's idea of what constitutes a "serving" or a "portion" can often be wildly different from yours, so adjust accordingly. Labels on cans or bottles of drinks often list the sugar content under "per 100 ml". However, a standard can is around 330 ml, which means you need to multiply the sugar "per 100 ml" figure by 3.3. If you don't do this, you'll be seriously underestimating how much sugar you're consuming.

THE ONE EXCEPTION: DAIRY

Whole milk (cow, goat or sheep) contains 4.7 g of sugar per 100 ml, meaning there are over 11 teaspoons of sugar per litre! However, the sugar in milk is a naturally occurring sugar called lactose, which our bodies can break down into glucose and galactose. Milk is therefore fructose-free.

This means that when you're working out how much sugar is in a milk drink, you can ignore the first 4.7 g of sugar per 100 ml. You can safely assume that any figure over 4.7 g is added sugar. For example, if your child's favourite chocolate milk drink contains 13 g of sugar per 100 ml, you know there is 8.3 g of added sugar per 100 ml (13 g – 4.7 g of lactose = 8.3 g). To convert this into teaspoons, divide 8.3 g by 4.2 and you know the drink contains 1.9 teaspoons of added sugar.

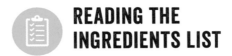

READING THE INGREDIENTS LIST

A quick way to check a product for added sugar is to read the ingredients list. Manufacturers don't like to make this too easy for us – they sneak sugar into their products in various guises. Did you know there are now more than 60 different names for sugar used in processed food? Here are some of the different types of sugar to look out for:

- Agave syrup or nectar*
- Barley malt
- Beet sugar*
- Blackstrap molasses*
- Brown sugar*
- Cane crystals*
- Cane sugar*
- Cane juice*
- Caramel*
- Caster sugar*
- Coconut sugar or coconut palm sugar*
- Corn syrup
- Demerara sugar*
- Dextrin
- Dextrose (another name for glucose)
- Fruit juice concentrate (often grape, as it's so sweet)*
- Fructose* (fruit sugar)
- Galactose
- Glucose (another name for dextrose)
- Golden syrup*
- High fructose corn syrup*

- Honey*
- Icing sugar*
- Invert sugar*
- Lactose (milk sugar)
- Malt syrup
- Maltose (malt sugar)
- Maltodextrin
- Maple syrup*
- Molasses*
- Muscovado sugar*
- Raw sugar*
- Rice syrup (or brown rice syrup)
- Saccharose* (another name for sucrose)
- Sucrose (table sugar)
- Syrup*
- Treacle*
- Turbinado sugar*

Common sweeteners:

- Aspartame
- Cyclamate
- Saccharin
- Stevia
- Sucralose
- Sugar alcohols: xylitol, maltitol, mannitol and sorbitol

* Contains fructose

WATCH OUT FOR THE FOLLOWING WARNING SIGNS

Sugar listed as the first or second ingredient – in an ingredients list, ingredients must be listed in order of weight, with the main ingredient first. If sugar appears as the first or second ingredient, steer clear.

Lots of different sugars – food manufacturers know we check to see if sugar is listed high up in the ingredients list and sneakily avoid having to put sugar as the top ingredient by using multiple forms of sugar and listing each one individually. As the sugar content is spread across several different types of sugar, they are used in smaller amounts and can legitimately be listed lower on the ingredients list.

"Syrup", "sweetener", or any word ending in "-ose" – as a general rule, if you see the words "syrup", "sweetener" or anything ending in "-ose", you can assume it's sugar.

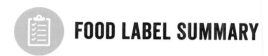 # FOOD LABEL SUMMARY

RULE 1: **Eat** products with less than 5 g of sugar per 100 g.

Stick to products that are less than 5 per cent sugar (i.e. less than 5 g per 100 g). If a product contains over 15 g of sugar per 100 g, it's a high-sugar food.

Remember: the maximum recommended daily intake of sugar is 6 teaspoons per adult per day.

RULE 2: **Drink** products with 0 g sugar per 100 ml.

That's not a typo! When sugar is in liquid form, its negative effects are magnified. The lack of fibre in the liquid means the sugar gets absorbed and sent to the liver very quickly, leading to fat storage and liver overload. The number-one thirst quencher to turn to is water.

TECHNIQUES TO BEAT SUGAR CRAVINGS

As you eat less sugar and your blood sugar levels become more stable, your cravings and urges to snack should start to disappear (along with other unsavoury symptoms, such as tiredness and mood swings). Your taste buds might undergo a similar transformation – foods you previously thought were bland may start to taste sweet and satisfying, and sugary food and drink, which you enjoyed before, may begin to taste super sweet. Here's how to start reducing (and eventually kicking) those cravings.

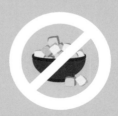

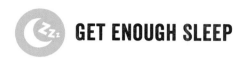 # GET ENOUGH SLEEP

Lack of sleep is like a mini hangover; it stresses the body and raises levels of the hormone cortisol, which fuels our appetite and increases cravings, particularly for sugary and carb-laden treats. The brain feels the full brunt of this energy crisis. A 2016 study found that a single night of sleep deprivation not only increased people's desire for junk food, it also increased the pleasure they derived from eating these foods. And that was just a single night – not days, weeks or years of chronic poor sleep!

A single good night's sleep can restore your brain to its optimal functioning. But how much sleep is enough? Everyone has different needs, but 7–8 hours is about right for most people. To optimize your sleep, avoid caffeine after 4 p.m. and switch off all your screens for a couple of hours before bed.

EAT PLENTY OF PROTEIN AND HEALTHY FATS

If you eliminate sugary food from your diet but don't replace it with nutritious and satisfying alternatives, your body's stress response will kick in, cortisol levels will be raised, and you'll be overcome with an irresistible urge to find a quick source of energy (high-fat, high-sugar food) as soon as possible. The trick to successfully reducing your sugar intake is to never let your body feel like it's being denied. The best way to do this is to eat "logs" (proteins and fats) rather than "twigs" (sugars and processed carbs).

Eating sugary food and processed carbohydrates (e.g. white flour) is like putting dry twigs on an open fire – they flare up quickly but don't burn for long (i.e. you feel hungry soon after eating them). Fats and proteins, on the other hand, are like logs on your metabolic fire – they take longer to get going, but they burn for hours.

If you add protein (some pieces of chicken, say) and fat (avocado and olives) to a salad, all of a sudden you have transformed your lacklustre dish into a tasty, satisfying experience. Use this trick with every meal and you'll be amazed how quickly your cravings diminish.

Healthy fats: Avocados, oily fish, coconut and coconut oil, hemp oil, olives and olive oil, nut oils (unheated).

Healthy proteins: Eggs, nuts, cheese (cow, sheep or goat), full-fat yogurt and Greek yogurt, meat and poultry, fish and seafood, grains and pulses.

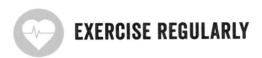 # EXERCISE REGULARLY

Exercise really is your secret weapon when it comes to stabilizing your blood sugar levels. Just 15 minutes on a treadmill has been shown to reduce cravings.

Not only does exercise increase glucose metabolism and insulin sensitivity, but there's good stuff going on inside the brain, too. When neuroscientists look inside the brains of new exercisers, they find an increased number of cells in the prefrontal cortex, the area of the brain involved in decision-making. Exercise is an internal stress reducer, too. It lowers cortisol levels and releases feel-good endorphins. (It's as effective an antidepressant as Prozac and cognitive behavioural therapy.) There's even new evidence to suggest that exercise changes how we respond to the idea of food by reducing activation of the parts of the brain that are associated with food cravings.

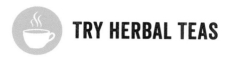 **TRY HERBAL TEAS**

Many herbals teas have a slightly sweet flavour, which can be soothing if you're craving something comforting. Try the following:

- Green tea
- Chai tea
- Spiced black tea
- Rooibos tea
- Cardamom
- Cinnamon
- Ginger
- Chilli

- Coconut
- Dandelion root
- Peppermint or spearmint
- Lavender
- Hibiscus
- Camomile
- Liquorice

- Cherry and cinnamon
- Orange and coconut
- Mixed berry
- Lemon and ginger

Note: Sadly, there's a proviso. If you regularly drink herbal teas containing fruit and citrus, there is evidence this can strip away tooth enamel. Herbal teas with no fruit content, such as camomile or peppermint, are not a danger to teeth. So use fruit teas occasionally and stick to herbal tea (or green tea, in limited amounts due to its caffeine content) for your daily consumption.

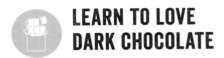 # LEARN TO LOVE DARK CHOCOLATE

In a low-sugar/low-fructose diet, there's no place for super-sweet chocolate bars. Switch to dark chocolate, which contains less sugar and is rich in antioxidants.

Raw cacao powder or nibs (little bits) – Cacao is different to cocoa, which may be sitting in your kitchen cupboard as hot chocolate powder. Raw cacao is made by cold-pressing unroasted cocoa beans so that the living enzymes stay in the bean and the fat (cocoa butter) is removed. Raw cacao is rich in minerals and potent antioxidants. It's also less than 1 per cent sugar. This gives you a clue as to how it tastes (it's pretty darn bitter). You can soften the taste by mixing it with other ingredients.

70–85 per cent cocoa dark chocolate – After raw cacao, the next best option is dark chocolate. Dark chocolate is rich in minerals such as iron and magnesium, but proceed with caution: it also has added fat and sugar. Look for a bar that is organic, free of additives, and ideally lists cocoa butter as the only fat. Stick to 70–85 per cent bars (85 per cent contains the least sugar), and savour just one or two squares at a time.

Sugar-free chocolate – Health food shops are overflowing with sugar-free chocolate. However, many bars are sweetened with agave, which is up to 90 per cent fructose, or maltitol, which is a sugar alcohol that the body can't digest properly. Stick to raw cacao or 85 per cent dark chocolate.

Home-made chocolate spread – Try mixing raw cacao powder with cashew nut butter (or another unsweetened nut butter) to make a delicious spread. Adjust the quantities to suit your taste.

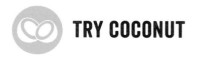 # TRY COCONUT

Coconut is a highly nutritious source of energy, packed with fibre, vitamins and minerals. It's easily digested, doesn't cause an insulin spike, its fatty acids (the good type) are converted into energy rather than stored as fat, and to top it all off, it's virtually fructose-free. What's not to like?

Whole coconut makes a healthy snack, and flaked or desiccated coconut is great sprinkled on desserts or into curries. Coconut water (if it's 100 per cent natural, with no added sugar or preservatives) makes a refreshing drink – try blending it with a handful of berries and some lime juice.

Coconut oil is one of the best oils to cook with, and coconut butter can be used in stir-fries or spread on pancakes. Coconut milks and cream are perfect for curries and making desserts.

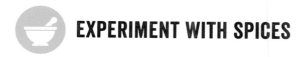 # EXPERIMENT WITH SPICES

Spices such as cinnamon, nutmeg, cloves, cardamom and coriander can "sweeten" food without adding sugar. Cinnamon in particular is a useful addition to your spice rack, as research suggests it reduces sugar cravings and stabilizes blood sugar. Use at least half a teaspoon per meal or drink:

- Add to muesli or porridge
- Sprinkle over warm almond milk, coffee or smoothies
- Add to stewed or baked fruit
- Sprinkle over fruit and yogurt desserts

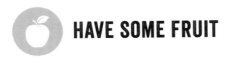 # HAVE SOME FRUIT

Yes, fruit contains fructose, but you'll also benefit from all the fibre, vitamins and minerals. Mix things up a bit. This makes sense from a nutrient point of view, too – different fruits contain different nutrients.

Given the choice of a piece of fruit or a standard chocolate bar, the fruit wins hands down in terms of healthy eating. However, if you suffer from cravings, it's a good idea to focus on savoury snacks like nuts over fruit, as sweet-tasting snacks can fuel sugar cravings. If you eat fruit between meals, eating it with something alkaline, like a piece of cheese, can help to protect your teeth.

TRY SWEET VEGETABLES

When sugar cravings hit, reach for vegetables instead. Starchy vegetables – such as potatoes, sweet potatoes and butternut squash – raise blood sugar levels more than non-starchy vegetables, such as broccoli, cauliflower and green beans, but they contain important vitamins and minerals. Root vegetables are naturally sweet and are some of the most nutrient-dense vegetables you can eat. Some of the healthiest sweet veggies are listed below. Just eat them in moderation.

- Sugar snap peas
- Podded peas
- Sweetcorn
- Red pepper
- Cherry tomatoes
- Pumpkin
- Carrots
- Parsnips
- Beetroot
- Butternut squash
- Sweet potatoes
- Onion

GO NUTS FOR NUTS

Nuts are rich in protein, omega-3 fatty acids, antioxidants, vitamins and minerals and are energy-dense, making them the perfect food to ward off cravings. Some nuts taste sweet and creamy, giving the illusion of having a sugary treat. Try raw macadamia and cashew nuts and sweet-tasting nut butters.

Have a small handful of nuts a day (30–50 g). Eat a variety of nuts, so you get a range of nutrients – walnuts, Brazil nuts, almonds, hazelnuts, macadamias, pecans, pistachios, cashews and pine nuts. Peanuts are technically a legume and are best avoided or eaten in moderation, as they are allergenic and can contain dangerous moulds that produce aflatoxin, a potent carcinogen.

BREAKING HABITS

When was the last time you opened a bottle of wine and thought, "Mmm, I'll just have some celery and hummus to go with that"? Whether it's alcohol and crisps or a cup of tea and a slice of cake, habits underlie much of our sugar addiction.

Happily, you can train your brain to get better at self-control. The brain remodels itself based on what you ask it to do on a regular basis. Practise juggling every day, and you get better at juggling. Practise a little self-control every day and your brain gets better at controlling your impulses. If you take small steps to reduce your sugar intake and use some of the strategies below, you should find that your biological drive to eat sugar loosens its hold on you.

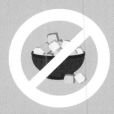

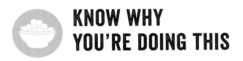 # KNOW WHY YOU'RE DOING THIS

The part of the brain that's in action when you succeed in resisting impulses and cravings is the prefrontal cortex. Its job is to steer us toward doing the right thing so that we achieve our goals. Knowing what you want and why you want it will make it much easier for your prefrontal cortex to do its job, to help you say "no" to the things that won't help you achieve your goal and "yes" to the things that will ensure your success.

To help you clarify a statement of intent around sugar, imagine how things will look in the future when your willpower is firing on all cylinders.

- How will you benefit from reducing sugar in your diet?
- How will your life change?
- Who else will benefit?
- How will you feel about yourself as you keep taking small steps and move toward your goal?

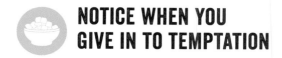 # NOTICE WHEN YOU GIVE IN TO TEMPTATION

The first step to breaking a sugar habit is learning how and when you give in to temptation. Chances are you don't eat cakes or crisps 24/7. Sometimes you can resist the urge and sometimes you can't. For the next day or two, simply notice what's going on. You might find it useful to keep a cravings diary for a week or so.

The second you realize you're about to give in to a craving for sugar, get curious. What's the situation? What's the environment? Who are you with? How do you feel? What are you thinking or saying to yourself that makes it more likely you'll give in to temptation? Does being worried or tired or overworked affect your choices? Did certain decisions help or hinder your willpower?

LIST YOUR SUGAR HABITS

Knowing when your willpower falters is crucial information because it means you can start to avoid the traps and triggers that herald an impending willpower meltdown. Start by making a list of all your sugar-eating habits. It's important to focus on the daily habits first, not the ones you do once a month or so. It might help to think about different situations.

For example, does being at the cinema make you think you want popcorn? Do you always grab a muffin or sugary coffee while waiting for the train? Do you reach for chocolates while watching TV, or when you're stressed? Are there always sugary snacks available at work? Does a certain friend always suggest getting a takeaway? Do you tend to snack when you're bored, or whenever you have a cup of tea?

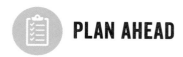 **PLAN AHEAD**

Once you've listed your habits, there are several ways you can begin to break their spell:

1. You can avoid the thing that triggers your habit.
2. You can replace your response to the trigger with a sugar-free alternative.
3. You can put an obstacle in the way of you and temptation.

All three strategies will require some planning and preparation, as explained in the next few pages. You need to be clear as to exactly how you're going to deal with specific sugar habits, so that you're ready to act when they crop up again in the future. Celebrate each time you stick to your guns; you are building new neural networks in your brain that will make it easier and easier to resist temptation as time passes. The key to creating "I don't need sugar" pathways in your brain is repetition. Keep at it, and things will get easier.

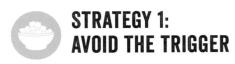

STRATEGY 1: AVOID THE TRIGGER

An obvious solution is to simply avoid the events associated with eating sugar altogether. OK, you can't cancel Christmas or ostracize your best friend, and avoiding events won't work on every habit, but it will for others. Here are some ideas:

- If you drive to and from work, take a different route and avoid the service station.
- If you walk to and from work, take a different route and avoid the vending machine or coffee shop.
- Shop with friends who support or share your low-sugar goals (and don't want to stop for coffee and cake).
- Avoid the kitchen at work when you know someone's brought cakes in – just don't go there!
- Switch to a different local café that sells healthy low-sugar foods.

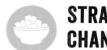

STRATEGY 2: CHANGE YOUR RESPONSE

This strategy involves keeping the habit (e.g. watching TV) but swapping your response (e.g. eating chocolate) for a sugar-free alternative. Make sure you have the alternative immediately to hand. You want to make it as easy as possible to switch. For example:

- When watching TV, have healthy snacks nearby, such as vegetable crudités or sweet potato crisps (see p.100).
- Replace the box of biscuits sitting next to the kettle with a jar of nuts and seeds.
- If you make a gin and tonic, swap the tonic for soda water with a squeeze of lemon.
- After finishing a project, give yourself a non-food reward, such as watching a favourite movie.
- Cut down on takeaways and make Friday night "home-made curry night", using fresh ingredients.
- Swap your burger and fizzy drink for a burger and bottle of sparkling water.

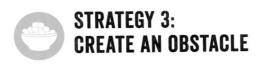

STRATEGY 3: CREATE AN OBSTACLE

One study found that simply placing sweets in an opaque jar, rather than a clear jar, on office workers' desks reduced consumption by a third. When the jars were placed 6 feet away so people had to get up to grab the sweets, consumption dropped by another third. Knowing this, you can tweak your environment in order to reduce temptation:

- Don't leave sugary snacks where you can see them. Out of sight is out of mind.
- Move temptations as far away from you as possible so you have to make an effort to get them.
- Get rid of temptation by removing all sugary snacks and drinks from your home or office space.

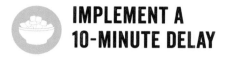

IMPLEMENT A 10-MINUTE DELAY

If you feel the urge to eat something sweet, like a Danish pastry for example, tell yourself you can have the pastry, but you need to wait 10 minutes first. Move yourself away from the treat, if possible, so that the reward seems less appealing to the brain. Once the 10 minutes are up, if you still want to eat the pastry, spend some time reflecting on why you want to cut down on sugar and the long-term reward you will gain by not eating the pastry. If you still want to eat the pastry, go ahead. By sticking to a 10-minute delay, you will be building your self-image as someone who can resist temptation and strengthening your ability to say no.

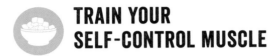 # TRAIN YOUR SELF-CONTROL MUSCLE

What's the best thing to do if your willpower is running low? Answer: pick a tiny aspect of self-control and practise it every day. Like a muscle, self-control gets stronger through regular exercise, and other aspects of your life will start to benefit, too.

Try implementing a tiny self-control practice every day for one week to get you started. Here are some ideas:

- Not eating sweets in the car.
- Writing down what you ate in your diary each night.
- Making your second glass of wine a spritzer.
- Eating half of a chocolate bar instead of the whole thing.
- Going for a 5-minute walk rather than drinking a sugary fizzy drink.

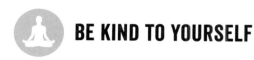 # BE KIND TO YOURSELF

Sometimes things go wrong. Let's say you have a bad day and eat a packet of digestive biscuits. You then feel so bad and consumed with guilt that you forget all the successful small steps you've taken up to this point and plunge into a vortex of overeating. "What on earth? I've had a bite of cake now, I may as well finish the rest of it."

The next time you suffer a temporary setback, talk to yourself as you would talk to your best friend, and offer support and encouragement. Your setback doesn't mean anything other than the fact that you are human. Your aim is to look after your health. You are allowed to falter. You don't have to be perfect. All that matters is that you pick yourself up and keep going.

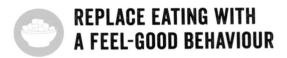

REPLACE EATING WITH A FEEL-GOOD BEHAVIOUR

According to American Psychological Association (APA) surveys, only 16 per cent of people who eat to reduce stress say that it helps them – the only reliable mood change they experience is an increase in feelings of guilt! The APA suggests we should ditch food and drink as pick-me-up strategies and turn to soothing feel-good behaviours instead. These activities trigger the release of mood-boosting brain chemicals, such as serotonin and oxytocin, in the brain. Strategies that are most effective at making us feel better include:

- Going for a walk
- Spending time on a creative hobby
- Exercising or sport
- Meditating
- Practising yoga
- Reading
- Listening to music
- Spending time with friends or family
- Having a massage

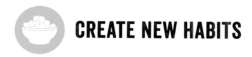 # CREATE NEW HABITS

Snacking is often a habit we've fallen into. Experiment with some of the new habits below and you should feel the pull of your old habits start to weaken:

- **Habit 1:** Be prepared. Take healthy snacks to work with you or keep some in your bag if you're out for the day.

- **Habit 2:** Replace tins of biscuits or chocolate with a jar of mixed nuts and coconut flakes (but stick to a small handful a day).

- **Habit 3:** Avoid snack-inducing behaviours. Instead of catching up with friends over tea and cake, offer to meet for a walk instead.

- **Habit 4:** Distract yourself. Go for a walk round the block, drink some water, hang out the wash, phone a friend or ask a friend or loved one for a hug.

MEDITATE BEFORE YOU EAT

Meditation alters brain activity and structure in several beneficial ways:

- It increases blood flow to the part of the brain (the insula) associated with awareness of bodily sensations, such as feeling full. Meditators have a thicker anterior insula.
- It increases the activity of the area of the brain responsible for decision-making (the dorsolateral prefrontal cortex), making it easier to choose healthier foods.
- It increases blood flow to the self-control hub of the brain (the anterior cingulate cortex), which helps us deal with impulses such as food cravings.

Next time a craving hits, try a 5-minute guided meditation (there are plenty of free apps available) and then see if the craving is still there.

ONLY EAT WHEN YOU'RE GENUINELY HUNGRY

Every day we rely on a host of external cues to tell us when to eat. We eat because other people are eating, because "it's time to eat", because we've completed an onerous task and are due a "reward", or simply because we're angry, lonely or bored. To tap back into your internal hunger cues, try the following:

- Ask yourself how hungry you are on a scale of one to ten. Genuine hunger is roughly seven on this scale.
- Check whether you're open to options. When people use food for comfort, they tend to crave a particular type of food (ice cream, chocolate, pizza), and only that food will do. In contrast, when we're genuinely hungry, we're more open to options.
- Tiredness can be a sign of dehydration. If you haven't had anything to drink for a while, drink a glass of water and wait for 10 minutes to see if you still feel hungry.

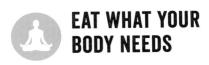

EAT WHAT YOUR BODY NEEDS

Studies show the brain lights up in anticipation of a reward, so the mere sight of a pastry or the smell of a baked cake can trigger the brain to release dopamine. Before we know it, we're speed-walking to the nearest shop (or our kitchen cupboard) for a sugar fix. Pausing for a few seconds can make a massive difference to your food choice.

Imagine you're having a chat with your stomach. Does it need something sweet or savoury, crunchy or smooth, light or filling? Picture some foods that fit this description. Imagine their taste, texture and smell, and most importantly, how you'll feel once you've eaten them. Keep "trying on" different foods in this way until you hit on something that feels perfect for your stomach.

As you keep practising the techniques in this chapter, you'll find it easier and easier to tune in to your body and differentiate "needs" from "wants".

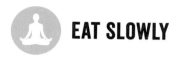 # EAT SLOWLY

It can take around 20 minutes for your brain to receive the message that your stomach is full. If you rush your food down in 5 minutes, the "I'm full" message will arrive too late – by this time you may have helped yourself to seconds or be reaching for a dessert. Slow down your eating and make sure you wait 20 minutes after finishing a meal before you even think about desserts.

FOCUS ON YOUR FOOD

If our minds are distracted, we miss out on the taste, texture and smell of food, all of which contribute to feelings of satiety. This is particularly important when eating sugary food. The next time you eat a dessert or some dark chocolate, try focusing 100 per cent on the experience. You should find, with practice, that you need to eat less before feeling satisfied. The following tips can help:

- Eat your meals away from any distractions – TV, phone, computer.
- Before you start to eat, really look at your food – all the colours, shapes and textures.
- Notice any feelings of impatience – any habitual urges to rush your food.
- While eating, see how many flavours and textures you can detect.
- Don't forget to use your other senses – notice the smell of fresh basil, the crunch as you bite into a carrot.

- Monitor how different foods "sit" in your stomach. Which foods make you feel alert and energetic? Which foods make you feel bloated, uncomfortable or sleepy?

- Notice how you feel an hour or so after eating. How's your energy? How does your stomach feel? How's your mood?

EAT UNTIL YOU ARE SATIATED (NOT STUFFED)

Eat until you feel satisfied, but not 100 per cent full (or "stuffed", to use a technical term). You can take your pick and visualize this as being anything between 70–80 per cent.

When nearing the end of a meal, focus on your stomach and gauge how full you feel on a scale of one to ten. Stop eating when you reach seven. Try using smaller plates and bowls. Food served on a small plate looks larger than the same portion served on a larger plate, so we feel more satisfied. Ditto for your wine or beer glasses – a tall, thin glass looks as if it contains more than a short, wide glass. If you feel the urge for a second helping, remember the 20-minute rule. Move away from the table and wait for a few minutes. This is easier to do if you've savoured your food.

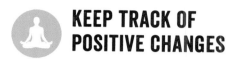

KEEP TRACK OF POSITIVE CHANGES

As you practise mindful eating, you'll notice your relationship with food changing. It's important to note (and celebrate) these changes in order to positively reinforce your new way of eating. This needn't be anything formal – make a mental note to yourself, share what you're discovering with friends or keep a journal and write a few words every day.

Here's a little quiz to help you get a feeling for how you're doing:

* Are you noticing how different foods make you feel?
* Are you tuning in to whether you're hungry, thirsty or bored?
* Are you slowing down and tasting your food more?
* Has eating become more pleasurable?
* How quickly do you feel satiated?
* Is it getting easier to make healthier food choices?
* Are your cravings diminishing?

A LOW-SUGAR DAY

Our busy days can be a sugar minefield. With long commutes, school runs, rushed or missed lunch breaks and evening plans (or just collapsing on the sofa), our biggest concern is time rather than nutrition: "What can I eat that can be prepared in seconds?" Add feeling tired or stressed into the equation, and our ability to make good food choices may be at an all-time low. Even if we opt for "healthy" food options to fuel our day, we can still end up feeling peckish and craving a sweet-tasting pick-me-up. Sugar lurks in the most unexpected foods – even the supposedly healthy ones.

This chapter will help you to identify some common sugar traps and give you some ideas and recipes for tasty, sugar-free alternatives.

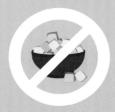

HEALTHY MEALTIME HABITS

To avoid rushing in the morning, get your breakfast ingredients ready the night before – put them on the kitchen counter or group them in the fridge so it's easy to grab everything as you leave the house.

Plan your lunches and add the ingredients you need to your weekly shopping list – if you have all the ingredients to hand, you'll be less likely to abandon your efforts and succumb to convenience food.

Make or prepare as much as possible the night before (e.g. a salad to which you can add a dressing and nuts the next morning before you head off to work).

Freeze soups and stews in individual portions and take them out at night to defrost so they're ready for the next day.

BREAKFAST: SUGAR TRAPS

We'll get the bad news out of the way first by looking at where hidden sugar lurks in our breakfast foods before moving on to the good news – quick, delicious alternatives that will help you start your day in a sugar-free way.

Table sugar – An obvious source of sugar in the morning is the granulated stuff you add to your tea, coffee, porridge or cereal. You may be using only a teaspoon here or there, but it soon adds up. Two cups of tea with a teaspoon of sugar in each, another sprinkled over your breakfast cereal, plus the five or so teaspoons hiding *in* your cereal... you could easily have eaten eight teaspoons of sugar before stepping out of the house.

Cereals – It goes without saying that chocolate cereals are high in sugar (most are around 35 per cent, or 4 teaspoons per 45 g serving). However, the figures for non-chocolate cereals are equally as shocking, and even so-called "healthy" cereals contain more sugar per serving than a jam doughnut (typically 10–15 per cent sugar and approximately 2 teaspoons per doughnut). When looking at these figures, bear in mind that the suggested serving size for most cereals is a miniscule 30–45 g, when most people have at least twice this amount.

Cereals that are marketed as being "high in fibre and low in fat" are often flakes coated in honey or sugar and mixed with dried fruit. Phrases such as "sweetened with honey", "no added sugar" and "natural sugars" are code for "contains fructose". Roasted and toasted cereals, such as granola, have sugar added to aid in the toasting. Many are 20 per cent sugar.

Low-sugar cereals – If you want to avoid the sugar traps, switch to low-sugar cereals, such as shredded wheat, wheat biscuits or sugar-free dried-fruit-free muesli. This small change can cut your sugar intake in one fell swoop. A 30 g serving of bran flakes can contain up to 2.4 teaspoons of sugar (assuming, of course, you stick to the 30 g). A serving of two wheat biscuits contains under half a teaspoon of sugar. Do this every day and you'll slash your weekly sugar consumption by 14 teaspoons! The best option of all is to make your own muesli – it takes seconds to make, you control the ingredients and it will store in an airtight container for several months.

Bread – I'm afraid there's more bad news about bread (I know; I wasn't happy about it either). Many shop-bought breads contain a surprising amount of sugar. Traditionally, white bread (4 per cent) and bagels (6.5 per cent) were the worst offenders, but recent analysis of some brown and wholemeal brands has revealed that many contain more added sugar than their supposedly inferior cousins, with some individual slices containing more than half a teaspoon of total sugars. Manufacturers say it's to "mask" the bitter taste of wholemeal flour, and the amount of sugar added is negligible – but, as we know, it all adds up.

There's an additional reason why bread is not your friend. As most of the nutritious part of the grain is removed in the milling process, all types of bread are rapidly converted to sugar once digested – even wholegrain varieties! The same goes for breakfast cereals. Opt for sourdough, rye or wholemeal pitta.

Spreads – Many jams and spreads are over 50 per cent sugar – you may as well spread a chocolate bar on your toast! (A bar of milk chocolate is around 50 per cent sugar.) Honey is about 80 per cent sugar, and even some sweetened nut butters, such as hazelnut spread, are 50 per cent sugar.

Your best bet is to go for unsweetened nut butters, such as cashew or almond (you'll find them in health shops and large supermarkets). Yeast extract spreads contain minimal or no sugar, but they contain high levels of salt, so spread thinly. Organic peanut butter is usually 2–3 per cent sugar. If you love peanut butter, it's probably best to eat it in moderation (rather than in spoonfuls every day). Or go totally natural and mash half an avocado with some black pepper and lemon juice and spread this on your toast.

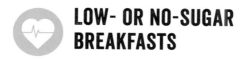

LOW- OR NO-SUGAR BREAKFASTS

If you've been eating the same breakfast every day for years, it can be difficult to imagine that an alternative exists. But it does – your taste buds just don't know it yet. A healthy breakfast containing protein and fat will fuel your body for hours, meaning fewer cravings and less of an urge to snack. Here are some ideas:

- Home-made muesli
- A handful of berries with nuts, yogurt and coconut flakes
- Porridge with cinnamon and berries
- Toasted sourdough or rye bread topped with half a mashed avocado, with leftover roasted vegetables
- Toasted rye bread with cheese and sliced tomato, black pepper and dried basil (under the grill)
- Coconut flour pancakes with berries and macadamia cream
- Vegetable and fruit smoothie (see p.90)
- Poached egg and wilted spinach or asparagus on sourdough toast with a knob of butter
- Hash made with leftover vegetables plus egg, cheese, fresh herbs and leftover tofu or meat

FETA AND SPINACH SCRAMBLED EGG

Serves 2

Ingredients: 5 medium eggs • 2–3 handfuls spinach • 100 g of cubed feta • Knob of butter or coconut oil • Black pepper

Wash the spinach and cook for 2–3 minutes in a saucepan until wilted, then drain. (There's no need for oil, as the spinach will steam in the water left on the leaves.) While the spinach is cooking, beat the eggs in a bowl and add black pepper. Melt a knob of butter or coconut oil, add the eggs and stir gently over a low heat until the eggs are almost scrambled. Add the spinach and feta and continue to stir for another minute or so. Serve immediately in a bowl – no toast required. For a fresh taste, try sprinkling with chopped chives and parsley.

HOME-MADE MUESLI

Makes one batch

Ingredients: 1–2 handfuls porridge oats or spelt flakes • 1–2 handfuls mixed nuts • Handful mixed seeds (e.g. pumpkin and sunflower) • Handful coconut flakes • Optional extras: 1 tsp cinnamon, 2 tbsp raw cacao nibs or 2 tbsp chia seeds

Mix all the ingredients together and store in an airtight container.

FOOLPROOF SMOOTHIE

Whizz up an item from each category for the perfect smoothie.

Liquid – Coconut milk, almond milk or coconut water

Vegetables (choose one to three) – A handful of spinach, watercress, rocket, kale or bok choy, ½ cucumber, 2–3 sticks of celery, or a small handful of parsley or mint

Fruit (choose one) – 3 strawberries, 1 handful of frozen or fresh mixed berries, ½ apple, ½ banana, 1 kiwi fruit, 1 slice of pineapple, or 1 pear

Protein (choose one or two) – 1 raw egg, 1 tbsp full-fat plain yogurt or Greek yogurt, 1 tbsp organic peanut butter or almond butter, or 1 tbsp nuts or seeds

Fat (choose one or two) – 1 small ripe avocado, 1–2 tbsp coconut (flakes or desiccated), or 1–2 tbsp hemp oil or coconut oil

Optional extras (choose one or two) – 1 tsp chia seeds, ½ teaspoon ground cinnamon or ginger, ¼ teaspoon of vanilla extract, 1–2 tbsp raw cacao powder, or a squeeze of lemon or lime

MID-MORNING MUNCHIES: SUGAR TRAPS

Cereal bars – Many energy bars, cereal bars and fruit bars have so much sugar they would be more at home in a sweet shop, with most containing at least 4 teaspoons of sugar. Check the ingredients list. "Sugar-free" bars usually contain fruit sugars from dried fruits like dates, which means they're packed full of fructose. If a bar doesn't contain fruit, it will be sweetened with something – honey, agave, maple syrup, cane sugar, artificial sweeteners.

Yogurt – Many single-portion yogurts contain at least 3 or 4 teaspoons of sugar. A yogurt with "no added sugar" may not contain cane sugar, but it will probably contain some other form of sugar. Avoid "diet" or "low-fat" yogurts. When manufacturers take fat out of their product, they put more sugar in to compensate for the lost flavour and texture. Low-fat yogurts often contain more sugar than ice cream (along with dubious synthetic sweeteners).

LOW-SUGAR SNACKS

Once you've been sugar-free for a few weeks, you should find that your urge to snack nose-dives – provided you are eating a combination of good-quality proteins, fats and complex carbohydrates, such as fruit and vegetables, to fill you up. Listen to your body. If you're genuinely hungry, eat something, but stick to real (unprocessed) foods. Here are a few ideas to get you started:

- Nuts
- A hard-boiled egg
- Olives
- A small piece of cheese
- Slice of smoked salmon
- Coconut flakes
- Home-made flapjack
- Celery sticks dipped in nut butter

- Vegetable crudités with hummus or guacamole
- Mini salad of mozzarella, tomatoes, basil leaves and olive oil
- Canned tuna or sardines with mashed avocado on sourdough toast

SNACKING FOR KIDS

Childhood is a time of rapid growth, and snacking plays an important part in meeting a child's nutritional needs. Here are some ideas for fun, healthy snacks:

- Ants on a log: Spread nut butter on half a stick of celery and dot nuts or chopped olives over the butter.

- Fruit and cheese stars: Use a small star-shaped cookie cutter to cut stars from slices of cheese and fruit (e.g. melon and apple).

- Orange and green chips: Roast sweet potato chips and serve with a green dip (mashed avocado with a squeeze of lemon or lime juice).

- Apple teeth: Spread two slices of apple ("lips") with nut butter and place chopped banana ("teeth") between the slices.

- Hedgehog hummus: Stick thin batons of carrots, celery and pepper in a small pot of hummus (add two raw cacao nibs or black olives for eyes if you're feeling extra creative!).

HUMMUS

Makes one batch

Ingredients: 400-g tin of chickpeas, drained
(or dried chickpeas, soaked overnight) • 1 garlic
clove, crushed or finely chopped • Juice of ½ a
lemon • 2 tbsp extra virgin olive oil • 1 tbsp
sesame seeds • Sea salt and black pepper

Blend all the ingredients together, adding more
lemon juice and seasoning to taste. Add some
water or a little more oil if the consistency is
too thick.

GUACAMOLE

Makes one batch

Ingredients: 2 large, ripe avocados • 1 garlic clove, crushed or finely chopped • 1 tbsp extra virgin olive oil • Juice of 1 lime • Sea salt and black pepper • Optional: finely chopped green chilli, tomato, red onion and coriander

Either blend all the ingredients together or, for a more chunky texture, mash the ingredients in a bowl. Add more lime juice, oil and seasoning to taste.

APPLE AND COCONUT FLAPJACKS*

Serves 8–10

Ingredients: 140 g rolled oats • 50 g desiccated coconut • 2 apples (seeds removed, unpeeled, chopped into quarters) • 2 tbsp chopped nuts (e.g. pecans or walnuts) • 1 tbsp honey (or sweetener of your choice) • 2 tbsp coconut oil • 1–2 tsp ground cinnamon (optional)

Purée the apples in a food processor with a tablespoon of water. Melt the coconut oil and honey in a saucepan, remove from heat and add the puréed apples and remaining ingredients and mix well. Grease a cake tin with a little coconut oil, and press the mixture into the tin. Bake in the oven at 180°C (350°F) for around 20 minutes or until golden. Leave to cool, then cut into slices.

*Note: These flapjacks do contain honey (a very small amount per slice), but they are far more nutritious than chocolate bars and most commercial cereal bars.

HEALTHY SANDWICHES

An innocent little cheese and chutney sandwich can contain 5 teaspoons of sugar. There's also the fact that bread is quickly converted into glucose in the body, so it raises blood sugar levels. Here's how to make your sandwiches healthier:

- Stick to low-sugar breads, such as sourdough, rye or wholemeal pitta.

- Where appropriate, omit the bread altogether and serve the sandwich filling on Little Gem lettuce leaves.

- Choose protein-rich fillings – such as tofu, tuna, egg or prawn – which balance out the meal and slow down the release of sugar.

- Get out of a sandwich rut by trying different ingredients – spinach, watercress or rocket, with shredded carrots, black olives, hummus and sliced avocado, for example.

- Watch out for dressings and sauces – especially pickles, chutneys, sweet chilli and hoisin sauce.

- Use low- or no-sugar spreads, such as mustard, olive oil, nut butter, tapenade, hummus, guacamole or yeast extract.

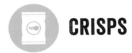 # CRISPS

Hang on, what have crisps got to do with sugar? Fat and salt might be a concern when buying crisps, but sugar is usually the last thing on our mind.

Most crisps are made from potato... and potatoes are a starchy carbohydrate... and carbohydrates get broken down into glucose in the body... and, well, you know the rest. The same is true for rice, corn (tortillas) and wheat (pretzels), too. Whether crisps are "natural" or not, and whether they are baked or fried, all will influence your insulin levels in a negative way. Remember:

- If you eat shop-bought crisps, eat them rarely (not every day).
- Crisps with the strongest flavours tend to be the highest in sugar.
- Steer clear of obviously sweet flavours, such as sweet chilli.
- Better yet, make your own crisps – then you can guarantee the ingredients.

KALE CHIPS

Makes one portion

Ingredients: 2 large handfuls kale • 1 tbsp olive oil •
Sea salt to taste • Other spices or seasonings to taste

Remove any tough stalks from the kale and tear
into rough pieces. Mix with 1 tablespoon of olive
oil and sea salt and any other seasonings to
taste. Arrange in a single layer on a baking sheet
and roast at 150ºC (300ºF) until crisp (around
20–25 minutes). Sprinkle with a little sea salt and
eat immediately.

SWEET POTATO CRISPS

Makes one portion

Ingredients: 1–2 sweet potatoes • 1 tsp
coconut oil • Seasoning to taste (sea
salt, chilli powder/flakes or cumin)

Thinly slice a sweet potato (keeping the skin on) using a potato peeler or mandoline. Oil a baking tray with coconut oil and cook at 200°C (400°F) for 10 minutes, turning halfway through. Season with sea salt, chilli powder or flakes, or cumin. Try roasting with sliced parsnips and beetroot for mixed vegetable crisps.

FIZZY AND SOFT DRINKS

If you've opted for a lunchtime meal deal, your sandwich and crisps might be washed down with a fizzy drink. Nearly four out of five carbonated, sugar-sweetened drinks contain more than six teaspoons of sugar per 330 ml serving. Seemingly healthier options, such as flavoured water, elderflower and traditional drinks like ginger beer and cloudy lemonade, contain more sugar than some colas. So, what can we do?

Don't drink them! I know that sounds harsh, but they contain nothing of any nutritional value, and they are one of the worst things for your health that you can consume. You would never pour yourself a glass of water and then add 6–12 teaspoons of sugar, but that's exactly what fizzy drink manufacturers do to every can.

Drink water instead. You can make it more exciting by adding fruit, basil, cinnamon sticks, ginger or mint.

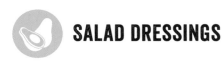 # SALAD DRESSINGS

Some salad dressings are not quite as saintly as they seem. Many contain more than 12 per cent sugar, which means that a 30 ml serving (2 tablespoons) can dump a teaspoon of sugar unceremoniously onto your lunch.

There's no need to shun salad dressings altogether – they taste good, and the fats help your body absorb the antioxidants in vegetables. Just switch to some better oil-based alternatives to help you get the most nutritional value out of your meal, or make your own salad dressing in seconds.

Use extra virgin olive oil or hemp oil as your base oil. Replace balsamic vinegar (high sugar) with unpasteurized apple cider vinegar, or red or white wine vinegar. Add garlic, herbs, mustard (wholegrain, French, Dijon), yogurt, and/or a squeeze of lemon, lime or orange juice, a pinch of sea salt and black pepper.

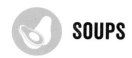

SOUPS

Soups can be a healthy option, especially if you make them yourself. Watch out for shop-bought versions, particularly tomato-based soups. Tomatoes contain natural sugar, but if slightly unripe tomatoes are used in soups and sauces, they can have an acidic taste. Sugar is added to soften this (the same is true of tomato sauces in baked beans).

Avoid canned products, as they have sugar added to extend their shelf life, and watch out for artificial sweeteners in low-sugar soups. Ideally, cook your own vegetable soup at home and freeze it in separate portions, ready for lunch during the week. Add meat, chickpeas or lentils to turn it into a more filling stew.

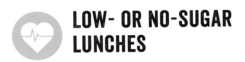

LOW- OR NO-SUGAR LUNCHES

There's no doubt that making your own lunch requires more planning than rushing to the shops and grabbing the nearest thing that jumps off the shelf, but making your own lunch puts you back in control. Here are some ideas:

- Generous salads using a variety of salad leaves, roasted vegetables, protein (fish, meat, cheese, nuts, seeds, boiled eggs), fats (avocados, olives, nuts) and a dressing
- Vegetable soup with added protein (i.e. meat, fish, chickpeas, grated parmesan topping)
- Hummus, grated carrot, pine nuts, coriander and rocket sandwich
- Vegetable frittata and salad
- Two cold chicken drumsticks with mustard, served with vegetable crudités and hummus
- Sushi
- Jacket potato or sweet potato with hummus or flaked mackerel and lemon crème fraiche

HOME-MADE SALAD DRESSING

Makes 180 ml (around half a jam jar)

Ingredients: 60 ml apple cider vinegar • 120 ml extra virgin olive oil • Pinch of salt and pepper • Optional extra flavours: 1 tsp Dijon mustard • ½ tsp honey or brown rice syrup • ½ clove of garlic, crushed • Pinch of dried herbs, such as oregano, marjoram or tarragon • Chopped fresh herbs, such as parsley, mint, chives or basil

Pour the above ingredients into a clean jam jar, shake well and store in the fridge for up to a week.

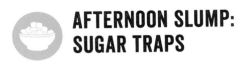

AFTERNOON SLUMP: SUGAR TRAPS

If you find yourself running out of steam halfway through the afternoon, it could be due to a number of things. It could be that you ate lots of sugary food earlier in the day and are on the sugar roller coaster, hurtling downward toward a dip. It could be the fact that you didn't sleep well the previous night, and your appetite control mechanisms are out of whack. Or it could be due to your body temperature dipping between 2 p.m. and 4 p.m. as part of your 24-hour cycle or circadian rhythm. Regardless of the cause, there's one end result: by mid-afternoon we feel tired and sluggish, and a sugary cup of tea with biscuits seems like a remarkably good idea. But this is the opposite of what our body needs. Sugary snacks give us a short burst of energy – and before we know it, we're heading for another energy slump.

Biscuits, cakes and chocolate bars – Coffee and a biscuit, tea and a slice of cake... hot drinks often trigger some of our worst sugar habits. Here are some biscuit guidelines to follow:

- Beware of "low-fat" or "diet" biscuits. Biscuits with reduced fat taste like cardboard, so manufacturers up the sugar content to add flavour.
- To reduce your sugar intake, you could switch to a savoury biscuit, such as oatcakes or multigrain crackers topped with plain butter, salmon, tuna, cheese or nut butter. (Remember the insulin response though; these are carbohydrates).
- The healthiest option is to ditch the biscuits, cakes and bars and make your own home-made bars or switch them for a healthy snack.

Hot drinks – One of the problems with buying sweet drinks from a café or canteen is that you'll have very little idea of what's actually in them – unless, that is, you happen to buy your drink from a high-street chain that posts its nutritional data on its website. A Starbucks grande cappuccino has 2½ teaspoons of sugar, and a chai tea latte has 10. Try these tips to reduce your sugar intake:

- Either go cold turkey and resolutely refuse to add any sugar to your tea or coffee, or take the small-steps approach and gradually reduce the amount you add each day in order to give your taste buds time to adjust.
- If you buy your hot drinks in a high-street coffee shop, take a look at the nutritional information listed on their website and switch to a low-sugar drink, e.g. replace your white chocolate mocha with a standard mocha – obviously, this doesn't mean the drink is good for you; just that you're reducing your sugar intake!

- As you would expect, the best options to go for are the plainest teas and coffees (fresh filtered coffee, Americano and espresso).

- Try sprinkling cinnamon on your cappuccino instead of sugar. Cinnamon helps stabilize blood sugar levels and adds flavour without the sweetness.

- Swap sugary hot drinks for sweet-tasting herbal teas, such as chai, vanilla, cinnamon and cardamom.

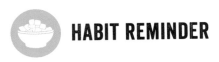 # HABIT REMINDER

The following healthy habits will help you ward off a mid-afternoon slump:

- Include protein-rich foods in your breakfast and lunch. This will help to fill you up and keep you going through the afternoon.
- Get outside at lunchtime and stretch your legs – the movement and exposure to natural light will refresh you for the afternoon.
- Keep your fluid levels topped up. Dehydration causes drowsiness. Don't wait until you're thirsty to have a drink because by then you are already dehydrated.
- Get up and move. If you work in an office, get up from your desk at least once an hour. Schedule physical chores for the afternoon – you could walk to the post office or shops, for example.
- Consider a standing desk.
- Stretch. Stretching limbs stimulates the brain and reinvigorates us.

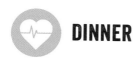 # DINNER

Have you ever come home at the end of the day and felt so tired (or stressed) it seemed like a monumental effort just to decide what to eat for supper, let alone physically prepare anything? Exhaustion, combined with work pressures and family commitments, makes takeaways and ready-made meals tempting options, but many contain high levels of sugar and have dubious nutritional content. (And that's being diplomatic. A study by the *BMJ* (*British Medical Journal*) analyzed 100 supermarket store-brand ready meals and found that none of them complied with nutritional guidelines set by the World Health Organization.)

Making the effort to cook a heathy, sugar-free dinner is the best possible option and doesn't have to be a big chore.

LOW- OR NO-SUGAR DINNER IDEAS

The ideas below all make speedy weekday evening meals. One-pot dishes, such as curries, pies and stews, are perfect for saving on washing-up and great for making in bulk and then freezing.

- Pork or lamb chop with stir-fried garlicky spring greens
- Marinated chicken breast (lemon and pepper) served with sweet potato chips and kale
- White fish fillet baked with green pesto and sliced lemon, served with steamed green vegetables
- Salmon fillet topped with red pesto, cherry tomatoes and black olives, served with green beans
- Vegetable or meat curry
- Vegetable stew (with seafood or fish, optional)
- Fish pie
- Home-made pizza
- Chinese stir-fry or broth
- Thai curry (add sugar-free Thai green curry paste to coconut milk and cook with sliced red pepper, courgette, baby sweetcorn, chestnut mushrooms, green beans, lime and coriander)
- Baked sweet potato topped with hummus and parsley, served with a salad

HEALTHIER TAKEAWAYS

A *Which?* study of Chinese, Indian and pizza takeaways found that Chinese takeaways contained nearly three times as much sugar as an Indian meal. The average chicken tikka masala contains 8 teaspoons of sugar, while the average Cantonese sweet-and-sour chicken contains an incredible 16 teaspoons. That's not including any sugar that will be converted from the carbohydrates in the fried rice. And let's not mention the fat, salt and food colouring content.

Pizzas contained the least sugar by far, but they still are made with processed flour in the base, which can cause blood sugar to rise rapidly. Stick to thin-crust pizzas.

Steer clear of obviously sweet meals, such as kormas and Peshawari naans, and sweet-and-sour or sweet chilli sauces. Low-sugar dishes include dry curries, such as tandoori with plain naan, and Chinese soups with steamed vegetables and prawns.

The healthiest option of all is, of course, to reserve takeaways for rare occasions and switch to home-cooked food.

MINI PIZZAS

Serves 1

Ingredients: 2 tbsp tomato purée (or home-made tomato sauce) • 2 wholemeal pittas • A few spinach leaves, wilted • A few fresh mint leaves, torn • A few black olives • Handful cherry tomatoes • Some feta cheese, crumbled • ½–1 clove of garlic, chopped • Salt and pepper to season

Smear the tomato purée or home-made tomato sauce on a wholemeal pitta and add 2–3 torn mint leaves and a few leaves of wilted spinach. Top with black olives, chopped garlic, cherry tomatoes and crumbled feta. Season with salt and pepper and pop under the grill for 5 minutes or until the cheese is lightly toasted.

CHEAT'S TOMATO SAUCE

Serves 2

Ingredients: 400-g tin of of chopped tomatoes
• 1 tsp coconut oil • 1 clove of garlic, sliced •
Handful fresh basil • Salt and pepper to season

Gently fry the sliced garlic in a little coconut oil for
1–2 minutes. Add a tin of chopped tomatoes and
a handful of torn basil leaves (or dried basil) and
simmer gently until the sauce has reduced. Add
sea salt and pepper and serve. You can make this
in big batches and freeze it in portions.

CAULIFLOWER PIZZA BASE

Serves 2

Ingredients: 1 medium cauliflower •
1 egg • 100 g goat's cheese or grated
cheddar • Salt and pepper to season

Grate a medium-sized cauliflower, cook in boiling water for a few minutes, drain well and mix with 1 egg, 100 g of goat's cheese or grated cheddar cheese and some salt and pepper. Shape the mixture into bases (roughly 1 cm thick), place on baking paper and bake for 30 minutes at 180°C (350°F) until golden and firm. Add your favourite topping and bake for 8–10 minutes. As an alternative, you can use baked portobello mushrooms or sliced aubergines for your base.

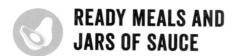

READY MEALS AND JARS OF SAUCE

Analysis by *Which?* revealed that many supermarket ready meals contain up to 10 teaspoons of sugar. Sweet-and-sour chicken with rice has up to 12 teaspoons of sugar and chicken pad thai with rice noodles contains up to 9 teaspoons.

Many shop-bought sauces also contain added sugar. Barbecue sauce has 3 teaspoons of sugar per 125 g, and a tomato and herb pasta sauce contains 2 teaspoons of sugar per 100 g. The figures may not seem too bad at first glance, but bear in mind that most of us don't use a 100 g serving of pasta sauce; we use 2–3 times this amount.

Always check the label and the list of ingredients, and beware of the "portion" size. If you eat a whole pack that claims it has 2 servings, you'll need to multiply the sugar "per serving" figure to calculate your true sugar intake.

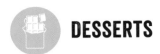 # DESSERTS

When we eat sugar, the brain releases dopamine, a feel-good neurotransmitter. High-sugar and high-fat foods work a little like heroin, opium and morphine in the brain, overwhelming our ordinary biological signals that control hunger. That's why people choose cheesecake over fruit salad.

At home, serve desserts in smaller bowls – this makes the portion look larger and can help fool the brain into thinking you've eaten more than you have. Switch to fresh desserts based on fruit and yogurt – a handful of chopped fruit topped with yogurt, coconut flakes, toasted walnuts and a sprinkle of cinnamon. In restaurants, swap dessert for coffee or a cheese platter, or go for a starter and a main rather than a main and a dessert. Try drinking a sweet-tasting herbal tea to quell any urges for something sweet to eat.

BERRY ICE CREAM

Serves 2

Ingredients: 2 handfuls frozen or fresh berries •
A splash of almond milk • A spoonful of nut butter

Blend all the ingredients, tip into a plastic tub and
place in the freezer for 2–4 hours.

CHOCOLATE MOUSSE*

Serves 2–3

**Ingredients: 2 very ripe avocados •
2 tbsp raw cacao powder • 1 tsp of honey
(or a sweetener of your choice)**

Blend all the ingredients and add more cacao powder or honey as needed. Try adding different flavours, such as the zest and juice of one orange or a few drops of vanilla extract.

*Note: It goes without saying that any recipe containing sweeteners, such as honey and dates, should be consumed in moderation.

COCONUT PANCAKES

Makes 6

Ingredients: 2 eggs • 2 tbsp coconut oil • 5 tbsp coconut milk • ¼ tsp salt • 2 tbsp coconut flour • ¼ tsp baking powder • Seeds and fruit to taste

Mix everything but the seeds and fruit into a batter using a blender or hand mixer. Let the mixture stand for 5 minutes to thicken. Stir the seeds and fruit (blueberries and raspberries work well) into the mixture. Lightly fry a tablespoon of the batter for each pancake. Serve with macadamia cream and/or berry sauce.

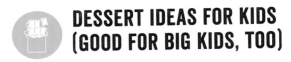

DESSERT IDEAS FOR KIDS (GOOD FOR BIG KIDS, TOO)

These fun, low-sugar desserts take just minutes to make:

Mango and coconut ice lollies – Blend one ripe mango with the juice of one lime and a tin of coconut milk. Pour into lollipop moulds and freeze.

Knickerbocker Glory – In a tall glass, layer fresh blueberries and raspberries with Greek yogurt mixed with desiccated coconut. Top with chopped nuts and a drizzle of honey.

Banana sundae – Chop a banana and add scoops of berry ice cream (see recipe on p.119). Top with coconut flakes and a drizzle of good-quality melted chocolate.

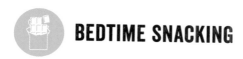

BEDTIME SNACKING

Snacking on sugars and grains before bed raises blood sugar levels. At some point during the night, they will come crashing back down again, which can wake you up or leave you tired the next day.

Try to wean yourself off your pre-bedtime snack habit. If you really need to eat something and/or hunger is disrupting your sleep, a handful of nuts and seeds can be a good choice, as they contain L-tryptophan, which promotes the production of serotonin, a neurotransmitter that becomes melatonin as darkness triggers sleep. Tryptophan is found in most protein-based foods – eggs, poultry, meat, fish and cheese. Try a pear dipped in hazelnut butter or a smoothie made from a third of a banana with some coconut milk and a tablespoon of nut butter. Camomile tea can also have a mild, sedative effect.

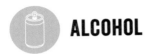 **ALCOHOL**

If your Achilles heel is a glass of wine or beer, you'll be relieved to discover that alcohol need not be banished altogether. You may simply want to tweak your drinking habits to ensure you're sipping less sugar.

A survey of drinks conducted in 2014 found that a certain well-known Irish cream liqueur contained the highest concentration of sugar (5 teaspoons per 100 ml), followed by sherry and cider. Dessert wines, fruit cocktails and sweet liqueurs were also rich in sugar. In contrast, most of the wines, beers and champagnes analyzed contained less than a teaspoon of sugar per glass.

In terms of sugar content, wine, beer and spirits are good choices, as most of the natural sugars in fruits, grains and berries are converted to alcohol during the fermentation and distillation process. Dry cider is better than sweet, but it does contain more sugar than wine, beer or spirits.

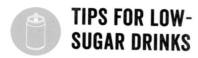

TIPS FOR LOW-SUGAR DRINKS

- The drier the wine or cider, the better.

- Red wine tends to retain less fructose than white.

- Beers contain maltose, not fructose, which is fine for us to digest (though some lagers and ales have added sugar or honey for additional flavouring, so always check the nutritional information on the bottle).

- Champagne isn't a great option, as it tends to retain more fructose.

- When drinking sparkling wine and Champagne, go for extra dry, brut or extra brut (extra brut is the driest).

- Beware of mixers, such as tonic water and fruit juice, which can contain 8–10 teaspoons of sugar in one tall glass. Drink your spirits neat (in small quantities!) or mix with soda water instead.

- Avoid flavoured drinks, such as ciders sweetened with cherry or raspberry.

CONCLUSION

Reducing sugar in your diet is not about being harsh or strict with yourself. Analyzing every morsel of food that passes your lips is not a recipe for health and happiness. Nobody wants to be celebrating a birthday or anniversary with a solitary cupcake shared between family and friends! The occasional sweet treat isn't going to undo all your good work if you're eating a balanced diet. What matters most is what you do on a day-to-day basis.

If swapping your high-sugar breakfast cereal for a low-sugar option feels achievable and easy, that's a great place to start. If trying a mindful eating technique feels exciting, that's the right small step for you. Small steps can seem inconsequential to begin with, but they soon add up. Consider the following:

- Swapping your morning glass of juice for herbal tea saves you 8 teaspoons of sugar.
- Swapping a shop-bought cereal bar for a handful of nuts saves 3 teaspoons.

- Swapping your can of fizzy drink for a glass of sparkling water saves 8 teaspoons.
- Swapping your ready-made meal for a home-cooked version saves 5 teaspoons.

These changes add up to 24 fewer teaspoons of sugar a day. That's 168 teaspoons a week! And that's just four changes – the tip of the iceberg.

Take a small step. *Celebrate!* Repeat. Get up the next day and do it again.

It's like the old Buddhist saying: "If you're facing in the right direction, all you have to do is keep walking."

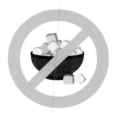

If you're interested in finding out more
about our books, find us on Facebook at
Summersdale Publishers and follow
us on Twitter at @Summersdale.

www.summersdale.com

IMAGE CREDITS